Where Is My Wife and What Have You Done with Her?

A Spouse's Guide to Her Menopause

Jeanne D. Andrus
The Menopause Guru

&

Jesse M. Andrus

Advance Praise for
"Where Is My Wife and
What Have You Done with Her?"

"Her body, her thinking, her emotions, her behavior — it all changes in a woman during menopause — but no one has thought to explain it to the men! This book is an essential guide for men to understand what's happening, what do to, and most important, what not to do to keep and reignite love in the next phase of their marriage."

Dmitri Bilgere
Author of "Beyond the Blame Game" and "Gateways to God"

"Jeanne and Jesse Andrus tackle not just what happens to a woman as she goes through menopause, but why it happens, combining biology, physiology and neuroscience (one of my favorite topics!) to explain why she's changing and how that affects a couple's relationship. As a relationship and intimacy expert for couples, with a background in math and neuroscience I have a particular lens to view the effectiveness of couples work, and Jeanne and Jesse are spot on with their creative and scientific approach that has the potential to refresh a tired relationship into a passionate, dynamic adventure together. I highly recommend this must have book for couples going through menopause."

Marla Mattenson
www.marlamattenson.com
Relationship & Intimacy Expert for Entrepreneur Couples

"As a Relationship Coach, one of the things that I teach all my clients is that research shows that the happiest couples understand each other's world. This book gives you a behind the scenes look at what's happening when menopause hits and how you can support your wife through it."

Maggie Reyes
Founder, www.modernmarried.com

JEANNE D. ANDRUS

JESSE M. ANDRUS

Dedication

To the men who seek to understand,
And especially to Jesse,
Who makes my days worthwhile
And lights up my nights,
Thank you for being you.
~Jeanne

To Jeanne,
Whatever comes,
it's my pleasure to be with you,
every day,
for the rest of our lives.
~Jesse

JEANNE D. ANDRUS
JESSE M. ANDRUS

Table of Contents

JEANNE D. ANDRUS

xii JESSE M. ANDRUS

Foreword

When it comes to the mysteries of menopause and the physical and emotional challenges menopause brings, there are lots of wonderful resources for women. However, there are not many resources for men to understand what's happening to their wives and their relationship with their wives during menopause, much less how to make it any better. And for that reason, this is an important book.

I met Jeanne almost three years ago, as we were working with the same publisher and in the same business mentorship group. But more than that, we also shared a love of serving women later in their lives. She was an expert on menopause and how to overcome its challenges in order to thrive again as a woman, and I was helping women in their struggling and disconnected marriages in their empty-nest years.

During the menopause years, of course, women experience countless physical changes, but they're also changing emotionally. They're shedding things that no longer serve them and awakening new desires that were kept dormant for many years. They're expressing their needs and making themselves a priority, which sometimes makes others around them feel like a lesser priority. These women are changing, and they're not going back to who they once were, making them unrecognizable to the men who have been by their sides for decades.

If this sounds like your beloved wife and your relationship seems to be growing increasingly distant, then it's time to understand what's going on before that distance becomes too far to bridge.

In this book, Jeanne and Jesse masterfully blend the science of what's happening with humor from a man's perspective to make the information easy to understand *and* the advice easy to accept – about what TO DO and what NOT to do – and apply in your life and your relationship with your wife.

This book is not written for women, with a few nods to men. This book is FOR MEN ... but not all men.

- This is for the man who wants to understand better what's happening to his wife and why she seems to be struggling so much right now.

- This is for the man who genuinely wants to make it better for his wife, to take away some of her pain, confusion or insecurities, while still allowing her to have her experience.

- This is for the strong man who is willing to do it differently with his wife in the second half of their lives: differently than he did throughout the first half of their lives together, in order to create a stronger, more communicative and connected relationship together.

By the end of this book, men will be equipped with a new understanding of how menopause is impacting their wives that will help them to make sense of the random and dramatic changes that seem to be taking over. Men will have real tools and suggestions of how to weather the storm for themselves, their wives, and their marriages. Although this isn't something a husband can simply fix for his wife, it is an experience that you can navigate together and come out the other side, closer than ever before.

In her book, *Goddesses Never Age*, Dr. Christiane Northrup, M.D. instructs us to "... make room for a partner if you desire one – or want to keep one." For men who take the time to read this book and are committed enough to apply its teachings, you are making room for your wife and her experience through menopause, as well as creating space for a new and improved relationship to unfold. And for women who share this resource with their husbands, you're making room for your husband to be a partner to you through one of life's great changes.

Sharon Pope
Master Life Coach on Love & Relationships and
Six-Time International Best-Selling Author

JEANNE D. ANDRUS

JESSE M. ANDRUS

Dear Confused-Husband-of-a-Unfathomable-Menopausal-Person (CHUMP):

Jesse speaks: Wait a minute, stop with the name-calling. This man is a CHAMP – Confused-Husband-of-an-ANNOYING-Menopausal-Person. He's not a chump at all!

Okay, we'll use Jesse's term for you....

Dear CHAMP:

You've probably wound up here for one of two reasons.

It could be that you're so confused by your wife's behavior and the symptoms she says she's experiencing, that you've gone looking for information about what's going on with her. Maybe you're thinking that all of these complaints and changes and upheavals are "all in her head," and you'd like to prove to her that there's a simple way to fix this. But I'd like to think that you arrived here because you care, and you're worried about the changes that you see occurring, and you want to do something to help her.

The other reason you may be here is that your wife is forcing you to read this book. She's tried to explain what's going on; she may have even said the word *menopause* (or one of its close relatives: *perimenopause* or *postmenopause*). But she's just out of explanations. She can't find the words that will help you understand (heck, half the time, she can't remember your name, so how could she explain *this*?). So, let's say she turned to me and asked me to help her explain to you what she's going through.

And so, here it is. The book is written for you – the confused person trying to understand why his life has been turned upside-down by what seems like it should be a welcome process. No periods? No more late night running to the drugstore for a box of tampons? No more PMS? No more fear of pregnancy or expensive birth control? It sounds like paradise to you, right? It seems like the two of you are right where you want to be – the kids are gone (or almost gone), the struggles are over, and the two of you can get it on anytime you want, right?

Not so. This person you're living with is decidedly not the person you married. From the woman who kept an immaculate house, did every chore with aplomb, and decorated for every season, she's gone to someone who's too tired and distracted to make sure that the dishes are in the dishwasher. And forget about making your dinner! She's telling you to make your own. And be sure to clean up afterwards.

She's gone from cuddling up to get her feet warm to sleeping in another room, chilled to an even -40°, and still she says she's too hot. Worst of all, she's absolutely not interested in sex. Says it hurts or she's not interested or even bursts into tears and asks how you could possibly be interested in her ugly body. She goes from laughing and happy to tears and rage in 0.4 seconds.

No, this isn't the person you fell in love with and married. This isn't the woman with whom you raised those wonderful kids. This isn't the woman you were so proud of at the company dinner as she smiled and applauded when you received that award you worked so hard for.

She must have been taken over by an alien. That's the only explanation.

The real answer is both more simple and way more complex than that.

Menopause is a natural process that occurs when a woman's reproductive system shuts down (over a period of years) because it no longer has any eggs to be fertilized. That's pretty simple, and, as I said, it should be a relief and the hallmark of a new and exciting phase of life.

Except.

Except that the hormones that make a woman all those things that we

JEANNE D. ANDRUS
JESSE M. ANDRUS

expect in a woman (and we women expect in ourselves) – caring, nurturing, efficient at running a household, and even interested in sex – also go away. We find ourselves not recognizing this person we are becoming. So it's no surprise that you can't understand her.

What I've done in this book is try to explain what is happening to your wife (in Part 1) and, more importantly, the response she'd like you to have (in Part 2).

Can I ask a favor?

I know that you're most likely a fixer – once you know something about something that's broken, you want to fix it (unless it's mowing the lawn or that toilet that won't stop running). Once you read Part One, you may think you have enough knowledge that you can just tell your wife what she should do and everything will be perfect again.

You won't. And it won't. In fact, you could make your situation a whole lot worse.

Before you do anything else, read Part Two.

Then, talk it through with your wife. Take the time to understand what she's feeling and how she would like you to act. See what her new view of your relationship is. And express what you're feeling now. Explain to her what you need in this relationship, not with ultimatums and angry words, but with love and understanding.

It's true. She's not the same woman you fell in love with and married. It's also true that you're not the same man she fell in love with and married. But the two of you can have a wonderful, loving, and supportive relationship for a long time to come, if you're both willing to do the work to create that relationship.

JEANNE D. ANDRUS
4 JESSE M. ANDRUS

Part One:
What's Really Going on with Your Wife

Hey, CHAMP.

This is where we talk about what is actually happening in your wife's body. The science – chemistry, physiology, and biology – of menopause. We'll talk about what that does to the way she thinks and feels, both physically and emotionally.

But don't think of this as a Chilton manual for that Corvette you want. It's not. I'm going to cover a lot of ground in a very short amount of space. It's an overview. It's like reading the owner's manual from the glove compartment – great if you want to know how to set the clock, but not so great if you're trying to tune the carburetor.

Jesse says: Don't think that just because you've read this part (or even both parts) that you have enough knowledge to jump in and "fix" anything. You just want enough information that you can nod and look wise. Trust me on this. Once you start trying to tell her what's going on in her body, she's going to give you "the look," and you're gonna wish you'd stuck with nodding and looking wise.

Just so you know, I talk about the underlying science in my books for your wife as well. I go into more detail there and on my website. Because she needs a

Chilton manual; you don't! You just need to get an understanding that this is real. Every bit of it is real, not in her head. In Part Two, we'll talk about how you can support her in creating her best body and life yet. Remember, though, it's always her choice to do anything. In this, you're here to support her.

Chapter 1
The Real Deal: What Happens in Menopause

Remember back in high school biology when learned about XX and XY chromosomes and how that was the difference between men and women? (**Jesse says: And then you went out and did some extra-curricular experimental biology and learned what the real differences are.**) If you're like Jesse, you may remember mostly the physical differences – breasts, vaginas, ovaries, penises, testicles. That stuff.

While it seems like the difference is in the equipment we come with, the physical makeup of men and women is only part of the story, and possibly not even the most important part of the story.

Jesse says: Wait! Go back! You mean, there's something other than breasts and V-J's???

Yes, Jesse (and you, Champ), there's a lot going on here. Stick with me for a little scientific tour.

What's Behind the V-J Curtain

Yes, Jesse, there is something else. How about a brief overview of a woman's "equipment," then? Here's a picture:

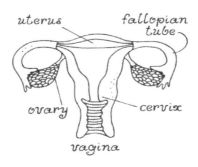

From top to bottom, we'll start with the *ovaries*. The ovaries are two glands on either side of a woman's *uterus*. When she's born, these are filled with immature *ova* (singular: *ovum*) or eggs (this is her whole supply; she never gets any more). Once she hits puberty, every month, one of these eggs develops and matures. When it's ready, it ovulates, leaving behind a sac that disintegrates and releases progesterone.

The ovum travels down the *Fallopian tube* to the uterus, where it may or may not be fertilized (that's where you and your swimmers come in). If the egg is fertilized, it can (but may not) implant into the lining of the uterus, where it develops into a baby over the next nine months. If not, the lining is shed in what you know as her "period" or *menses*. That happens, as you're probably aware, on roughly a 28-day cycle.

Just for completeness sake, the uterus has a semi-open sphincter separating it from the vagina, known as the cervix. Then there's the vagina, and its opening. Finally, most women would like me to remind you that outside the vagina is the *clitoris*, which is one of the chief pleasure spots for women.

Okay?

Jesse says: I knew that! Well, not really. But now I do.

Why Hormones Matter

Many of the differences in how men and women look, feel, and respond to the world come from the differences in their endocrine systems. *Endocrine system* is a rather loose term for one of the major communication systems of our bodies. It consists of hormones, neurotransmitters, and the glands that secrete them. Hormones are produced in various parts of our bodies and used to transmit statuses and trigger processes in various parts of the body.

The endocrine system in humans is highly complex (so complex that we're still discovering new hormones and neurotransmitters even today). It's also tightly coupled, meaning that what happens with one hormone can affect how, or even if, others work.

Perhaps the most important difference in the endocrine systems of men versus women is in the "sex" hormones that govern the way our reproductive systems work. Men's reproductive systems are driven by a group of hormones known as *androgens*. The most well-known of these is *testosterone*, but there are really three of them – testosterone, *aldosterone*, and *DHEA*.

Women's reproductive systems are driven by two hormones – *estrogen* and *progesterone*. These two hormones are produced in several places in their bodies, but the versions we really want to talk about are produced in the ovaries and uterus. Their production is driven by their monthly cycle.

Progesterone is produced when the ovum is released at ovulation and the sac that contained the ovum disintegrates. Estrogen is released slightly earlier in the cycle, as the ovum develops toward maturity. (Estrogen is also produced in fat cells, and both progesterone and estrogen are produced in the *adrenal glands*. This occurs in both men and women.)

What's important to know here is that, prior to puberty, young girls don't have much estrogen and almost no progesterone. Puberty, for girls, happens when the pituitary gland (an area of the brain) releases a signal to begin maturation of an ovum. While that ovum is maturing and releasing, estrogen and then progesterone are released.

This cycle continues, somewhat irregularly at first, and then settling in to a pattern of approximately every 28 days, except when a woman is pregnant or nursing, until sometime in her late thirties or early forties.

By then, the number of viable eggs has decreased sufficiently that one does not mature every month. When that happens, ovulation and the release of progesterone doesn't happen. Estrogen, though, usually continues to be released in this early stage of what's called perimenopause.

For many women, this is when they first begin to notice changes in their body, the way they think, and in their emotions. The symptoms of perimenopause are many and varied and can come and go throughout her journey through menopause. She, and even her doctor, may not recognize all of the symptoms as being caused by these hormonal changes.

The cycles which don't produce ovum (called *anovulatory cycles*) continue to happen more frequently. At some point, women may begin to skip their period, have extremely heavy periods, or have longer or shorter intervals between periods. Finally, ovulation ceases altogether, and so do her periods. After 12 months without a period, a woman is said to have reached menopause.

Technically, menopause lasts just one day. It's the first anniversary of a woman's last period. But don't get too excited. That just means that she shouldn't get a period again (and most doctors will say you two don't need birth control any more).

The day before menopause, she was perimenopausal. Now, the day after, she's postmenopausal. At first, her body will still be adjusting to the new levels of hormones and to the lack of a cycle. She may experience new symptoms, or some old ones may continue. For some women, the finality of this change may also carry some emotions, especially if they regret choices or circumstances around having children.

Just to recap about the hormonal changes. First, progesterone drops, while estrogen stays the same or possibly drops. These changes aren't linear – fluctuations seem to occur randomly, and sometimes within a very short period of time (minutes, not months). As perimenopause progresses, progesterone and estrogen levels drop and stay lower for longer periods of time. After 12 months with no period, a woman is officially postmenopausal, and her hormones begin to stabilize at very low levels.

Is That All?

You may be thinking that that doesn't sound like a lot. In fact, it may even feel like something you'd think women would welcome. After all, your wife may have been complaining about her period and the things that go with it (like PMS, migraines, bloating, and water weight gain) for years. She should be happy now, right?

It's not so simple. The problem is that estrogen and progesterone have been given other jobs to do in a woman's body. Remember I mentioned that the "parts" weren't the whole story when it came to the differences between men and women.

It turns out that these hormones play a role throughout a woman's body and brain in determining how she looks (things like skin softness, bone hardness, and hair growth), in how she thinks, and how she feels, emotionally. Almost every cell of her body has receptors for estrogen and progesterone, meaning that almost every cell will take in these hormones and use their levels as a signal, or use the hormone itself as a building block for one of its processes. As these hormones reach their new levels, she'll experience changes in every area of her being.

Then, there's the collateral effect on the rest of the hormones and neurotransmitters floating around her body. It turns out that hormones and neurotransmitters are often affected by other hormones and neurotransmitters. In particular, estrogen affects how women experience cortisol – the stress hormone. It also affects how women process blood sugar, making insulin resistance something they are much more susceptible to. And, it affects how thyroid hormone is used. Progesterone affects both serotonin, one of our "feel good" neurotransmitters, and melatonin, the sleep neurotransmitter.

In the rest of part one, I'll be explaining in general terms some of the changes that your partner may be experiencing or you may notice in them. But the more general truth is that menopause, with the changes in levels of estrogen and progesterone, affects every area of a woman's existence. Most symptoms she experiences during this time of her life may have a link to the changes in one or more of the hormones affected by menopause. I actually tell my clients to let any medical practitioner know where they are in their journey whenever they have to deal with a medical issue.

Chapter 2
Her Changing Body

As I've helped my clients with what's going on in their bodies, I've researched dozens of changes, symptoms, and side effects that are attributed to menopause. Your spouse may experience some of them, or not many of them at all. Some may bother her, others she may deal with easily, and still others may scare her or cause her no end of problems. It really is an individual journey, and what bothers one woman, another may scarcely notice.

Then, there's your side of things. You may notice a lot of changes. Some things about your "new" wife may not be so pleasing to you. You may want your old wife back (and I can assure you that there are probably times she wants her old self back again, too, as well as times she might be wishing for the younger you to return).

Jesse says: I just got confused. You mean menopause isn't the same for every woman? I really need a manual!

Changes happen in every area – body, mind, emotions, and what I'll call spiritual changes. Some of these will be apparent to you. Others will happen inside, or she may hide them from you. I don't want to list every symptom, because it tends to start people on a wild goose chase with thoughts like, "Do I have that symptom? Did I miss it? Maybe that weird feeling I had last Sunday was (fill in the blank)." What follows is a description of the kinds of things that she may be experiencing in each area.

There are a lot of changes that happen in her body. Some of them may be very like the things that are happening to you, too. They're really effects of getting older – things like graying hair and maybe wrinkles starting to appear (**Jesse: don't you call them wrinkles, though,**

CHAMP – call 'em fine lines, emphasis on fine). Some of them have to do specifically with her reproductive system; others feel unrelated to menopause, but are.

Fertility and Periods

Babies. Who wants 'em; who can have 'em? Here's the problem. With today's science, no one can tell beforehand exactly when a woman will stop ovulating. As long as she's ovulating, there's a chance she'll get pregnant with unprotected sex. One thing that's important to mention here is that among these "older ovum," there is a higher chance for congenital and genetic abnormalities.

There also seems to be a common pattern among the women I work and talk with, that sometime during late perimenopause, a desire for one more baby takes over our thinking. We daydream names and redecorate our college-aged son's room pink (in our minds) for the baby we think we want. We skip a period and run to the store for a pregnancy test, half in dread and half hoping for a positive result. If this horrifies you, don't panic. It's a hormone-triggered phase that passes fairly quickly. Just don't miss on the birth control, because together with the desire, there are hormones acting in the background that mean she's likely to be fertile at the same time.

Another note about birth control. It's most likely that her doctor will take her off any form of birth control that contains hormones as she approaches the final stages of perimenopause in order for her body to finish its transition. Therefore, some barrier form (e.g., condom or diaphragm) is needed.

Jesse says: Time to replace that old condom in your wallet. Make sure you have one that works.

Don't take chances, because as her fertility comes to an end, so has the regularity of her periods. Longer or shorter intervals and lighter or heavier periods are common, and if your spouse has symptoms associated with her period, like PMS (pre-menstrual symptom) or migraines, you may have been living in an unconscious rhythm with them. That will probably change and you may feel, consciously or un, the change in the pattern of your life.

Finally, there comes a time when it seems the periods have stopped. That may be right, or they may show up again. Unfortunately, it seems to be unpredictable, and, honestly, the problems that you have with this are nothing compared to her discomfort and discouragement.!

Weight Changes

Nothing – even our wonky periods – is as annoying to most women about the process of menopause as the change in weight. It seems to happen to most women. Either they gain weight and can't seem to lose it, or their "extra" weight shifts to belly fat, or, in a few cases, they lose weight and can't seem to keep it on.

We try, oh, we try. We try our favorite diets and fad diets. We head to the gym or out on the road, walking or jogging for miles. We moan to our friends and spend hours staring at the full length mirror this way and that. We make you join us in our diets and then are furious when you immediately lose five pounds, while we gain two.

Most of all, we hate our bodies. Even women with positive body images (almost nobody, by the way) find themselves angry, confused, and despondent over the weight changes that they can't seem to control. Even a tender touch can send us into a rage. It may feel like it's aimed at you, but it's really directed at ourselves.

Jesse says: You know that question, "Does this make me look fat?" If you haven't heard it before, you'll hear it now. There is no winning this one. I suggest a small box of dark chocolate, a glass of wine, and soft lighting.

Skin, Hair, and Nails

Yes, we're getting older (and so are you). The things that we think of as aging, happen. Our skin gets drier and fine lines (aka, wrinkles) appear. Our hair changes color – sometimes naturally, and sometimes because we spend hours at the hair salon with our colorist (that may be a new member of your household, but she's important to your wife!) restoring our natural color or trying out the latest trend (aqua, purple, magenta?) in hair colors.

Other changes are peculiar to menopause, and they're way more aggravating. One of the most annoying is the changes to our hair. For some of us, it migrates – from the top of our head (and sometimes, our eyebrows) to our chin and upper lip. While the "stray hairs" – the ones on the lip and the chin – are obnoxious, they're fairly easy to deal with. It's when our crowning glory, our hair, thins and falls out that we freak out.

Other symptoms we hate, and you should probably pretend not to notice, include acne (really?), brittle and breaking nails, and even changes in our body odor.

Beneath the Surface

There's no doubt that for those of us going through menopause, what we see when we look into the mirror is annoying and depressing. It clearly reminds us that we're no longer young. But what's happening underneath can be downright scary. Many of the physical symptoms we experience can seem bigger, especially if we're experiencing a group of symptoms. Then we call Dr. Google (a quack if there ever was one) and decide we have cancer, or exploding heart syndrome, or some other dread and impossible disease.

Unfortunately, that tends to result in appointment after appointment with specialists who look at only the symptoms that relate to their

JEANNE D. ANDRUS
JESSE M. ANDRUS

specialty. Test after test shows nothing, and they decide that it's all in our heads. We go home with a prescription for Prozac and a recommendation to call a therapist. So, now we're menopausal _and_ crazy.

And so it goes, until the next set of symptoms appears.

I could bore you with the whole long litany of symptoms. From anemia due to extended periods, to heart palpitations that have us rushing to the hospital in the middle of the night, to the feeling of ants crawling under our skin, the list is long, daunting, and discouraging. But even if I recited every item in that list, it's possible your beloved is suffering with something _else_ that doesn't seem like it's related to the hormonal changes of menopause, but is.

Here's the truth. If she's telling you something feels weird in her body, it probably really does. It's not made up. If she tells you she feels lousy, but she just can't describe it, that's almost assuredly true. If she tells you that she's experiencing something totally weird, like her tongue is burning or she feels like she's being shocked repeatedly, she's feeling that – those are real symptoms.

We'll talk more in Part Two about how you can help, but for now, I just want you to know two things. One: It's real. It's not all in her head and she's not crazy. Two: When she's seeking help, remind her (gently) that these may be symptoms of perimenopause or postmenopause, and if her medical practitioner doesn't recognize that, she may want to find one who does.

And _always_ tell Dr. Google that menopause is a factor.

JEANNE D. ANDRUS

JESSE M. ANDRUS

Chapter 3
Her Changing Thinking

Jesse says: I've got the changing body stuff. It even makes some sense. But what about all the crazy things you did? What about the bad moods and black rages? What about the anxiety and not leaving the house? What about the forgetfulness, and the disorganization? That's a lot harder to deal with than the physical changes!

To my great chagrin, I learned, when raising a boy, that the "we're all the same; it's all in the upbringing" rhetoric that pervaded my late teens was just not true. There are similarities, and for sure there is a spectrum of any given quality. But, girls are not the same as boys. And women are definitely not the same as men. And I'm not just talking about the physical stuff here.

A bit of background is in order. Back in Chapter One, I briefly mentioned that estrogen affects every cell in a woman's body. Some of the most important effects are those that happen to her brain, because the brain is the most important center for determining how she thinks, feels, and acts. Beyond the brain, there are also interactions between the hormones that change in menopause – estrogen and progesterone – and the other hormones and neurotransmitters that influence thinking and behavior.

Evolution used these interactions to create patterns of thinking that made humans as successful a species as we have been. We've been specialized to operate and think differently as men and women, so that we can raise the next generation safely – safe from saber-toothed tigers and famines.

Think about how women lived 10,000 years ago. They were often pregnant, unable to run or hunt. The young ones that were born would take several years to become independent, and a child who lost its mother was especially vulnerable.

Women needed the ability to create a family, a home, and a community to protect their children. That requires communication and cooperation, even-temperedness, and the ability to resist the urge to panic – to fight or to flee. Men, on the other hand, were most often the hunters and the warriors. Tracking and trapping required a different set of skills – more solitary and more spatial thinking. When danger was present, fighting or fleeing as a response made more sense.

Rather than develop separate physical structures to accommodate the differing needs of the genders, it was easier for our hormones to evolve to direct the show. Our differing hormones have hard-wired those roles, to some extent, in women versus men. And then menopause comes along and changes the hormonal balance.

It plays out in the way we think and feel in our reproductive years, and for women, changes how we think and feel as we enter and progress through our menopausal changes. In this chapter, I want to tackle how the way women think changes in menopause. Then, we'll look at the effect on emotions and her sense of self, and even changes in her sexuality in the remaining chapters of part one.

The Effects of Diminishing Estrogen

Estrogen stimulates a couple of key areas in the brain and creates a different experience of the world for women than the one you experience. It's probably made life with your spouse interesting and even problematic for years. You may never have known why until now, when it's changing and giving you a whole new set of problems to deal with.

The first area is one in the prefrontal cortex, which is the center of our higher thinking abilities. This area, the *frontopolar prefrontal cortex*, is responsible for what is commonly called multitasking, and it's powered by estrogen. It isn't really multitasking; women aren't a whole lot better than men at doing two things at once.

However, estrogen-driven women have an ability to go from completing part of a task to a different task and circle back to the original task. A common example is cooking. Let's say your (premenopausal) wife is making spaghetti sauce. She might chop the onions and peppers, set them to browning in a pan, run into the laundry room and turn on a load of clothes, stop and check on your five-year-old playing in his room, and return just in time to add the meat. She doesn't think twice about where she is in the process; she just picks up where she left off.

Now, without the estrogen stimulation, this ability isn't as reliable. She might not remember to return to the kitchen until she smells the burning onions as she walks by the kitchen (or the smoke detector starts screaming). Similarly, she might forget the now-wet clothes in the washer until you need your favorite shirt, three days from now. Now, this inability to move seamlessly from one thing to another and back might seem perfectly normal to you, but for her, she feels like she's losing her mind. She can't remember a thing and nothing ever gets finished. *Cue tears, anger, frustration.*

Then, there's the memory lapses. These happen especially around things your wife has always been pretty good at. Things like people's names, and pulling the right word out of the air when she needs it. You may have marveled at her ability to remember the names of the church members she only sees a couple times a year or the names of every one of your children's teachers. You may even rely on it to keep you from being embarrassed at parties when you forget your best friend's name.

The reason that women have such fabulous communication skills is that estrogen stimulates a secondary verbal area on the opposite side of their brains. Everyone, men and women, have a left-brain verbal center, but women in their reproductive years have a much more developed secondary verbal center on the right side of their brain. It's stimulated by, you guessed it, estrogen.

Then, the levels of estrogen drop and boom, that right-side verbal center is no longer receiving the same stimulation. And she's forgetting the name of her best friend and the word for the thing-ama-jiggie that opens the can that's got the what'zit in it. Once again, she's confused. More importantly, she's scared. Her Aunt Gerry started forgetting the words for things, and it turned out to be a brain tumor (or Alzheimer's). And even if she isn't scared by these "senior moments," she's embarrassed and angry and frustrated.

The Effects of Other Hormones

There are other changes in the way she thinks. There's a generalized "brain fog," which feels like all your senses are damped down. Feeling confused or scattered. The inability to concentrate. Feeling like your thinking has slowed down, or you can't connect the details. Does menopause create all these problems, or should she (and you) be worried about Alzheimer's?

Remember back in Chapter One, I mentioned that other hormones get into the act? Well, this is an area where imbalances in two hormones, in particular, can cause or exacerbate the symptoms. *Cortisol*, our primary long-term stress hormone, and *thyroid hormone*, which regulates our metabolism, can both affect the quality of our thinking when they are out of balance.

What this means for your wife is that she can pile up a whole lot evidence for her hypothesis that she's either A) going crazy or B) got Alzheimer's. Either way, those are scary propositions for her. And when they pile on to the other symptoms, she's likely terrified of what the future might bring.

Especially if cortisol, the stress hormone, is involved, the stress and fear is going to make it feel worse. And while you don't think these slips are a big deal (because that's the way you may have approached life all along), she does. It's different for her. It's never happened before.

Jesse says: In our house, it's just what we do. Jeanne asks, "Do you remember where..." and I say, "Let me introduce myself." Recently, she's started saying the same thing. The bad news is that we buy a lot of duplicate items because we can't find something. The good news is, that now that she understands it, we laugh a lot over these slips.

Chapter 4
Her Changing Emotions

Her brain is changing, and her body is changing, but I bet you haven't noticed any mood changes, right?

Jesse says: WHAT?

Okay, I'm kidding. Her moods are all over the place, changing moment to moment. Or she's depressed. Or anxious. Or she doesn't ever want to leave the house or talk to anyone new or even hang out at your sister's house with the family.

While you can understand that there are physical changes that affect more than just her reproductive system and you'll accept that maybe estrogen and progesterone have something to do with changes in the way she thinks, you wonder: how could those hormones affect her personality?

Does she hate you? Sometimes she seems so mad. It seems like you can't do anything right. Then, the next minute, she's sobbing and telling you how she can't do anything right and how she hates herself and that you're the best husband ever for putting up with her. Twenty minutes later, the whole thing's a distant memory, and she's wondering why you aren't getting ready to go to the barbeque at the neighbors.

And your head is spinning.

What's Going On?

The emotional effects of menopause are just as big as the physical effects and perhaps more perplexing, to you and to her.

Some of the more obvious things you might see are mood swings – changes in mood from moment to moment, depression, anxiety (sometimes accompanied by full blown panic attacks), frustration, and irritability.

These emotional changes arise primarily from the same place that all menopausal symptoms come from – from her changing hormones. The problem is that we are accustomed to viewing volatile emotional changes, anxiety, and depression as "psychological disorders." We immediately view ourselves as crazy, or, if we're more "civilized," in need of therapy.

So, let's look at a few of these symptoms and why and how they become common in menopause.

Anxiety.
I want to start with anxiety, because it's one of the easiest to understand.

First, let's separate anxiety into two parts. The first part is the fear or the worry, which could be about almost anything, rational or not. Fear, contrary to the oft-repeated adage "False Evidence Appearing Real," is the reaction to a perceived threat. Someone could be fearful about passing a test, about encountering a snake, or about driving to the store three blocks away after a bad experience the week before. Worry is a little less tangible. Worry is fretting over potential outcomes that may or may not happen. We worry about our children leaving home, what would happen if we lost our job, or whether we misplaced our wallet (even though we can't check in our purse right now).

The second part is the physical reaction. It arises from the adrenal glands with the release of two hormones – epinephrine and cortisol. It feels like your heart is racing, your breath is shallow and quick, you become hyperaware as you look for the threat. Your muscles tense, preparing to go into fight mode or to flee. You've probably felt this feeling many times in your life.

For your wife, though, for much of her life, her reaction to a fear stimulus has been different. Estrogen has dampened the physical reaction, allowing her to act in a more controlled way. When the fear happened, she considered her options, took care of the things (or the people) who needed caring for, and worked with her friends to fix it. It was only when the fear got massive that she felt that "fight-or-flight" thing. Without that estrogen changing the reaction, she'll start feeling cortisol that way all the time.

New scenario. Now, estrogen is low and cortisol is up (sometimes way up). Some little miniscule thing comes along to startle her or concern her and bam... she's over the edge. Anxiety takes over. Full-blown panic ensues. Because as a society, we attach anxiety to events, she looks around. What triggered it? She looks to find a cause. Whatever happened in proximity to it becomes the cause. And now the cycle starts. The next time the trigger is encountered the physical reaction happens, the trigger is more feared, and the reaction gets bigger.

Here's how that escalated for one of my clients. Denise had been tooling around her town for years, driving herself and the kids everywhere they needed to go. She'd missed 4 periods (meaning her estrogen was low), and she was juggling worry about a financial setback, tight deadlines at work, and her daughter's senior year. One day, she was thinking about her finances, and she found herself shaking and crying at a traffic light. Just then, she heard a car slam on its brakes nearby. Over the next few weeks, she got more and more nervous about driving in that area. Six months later, she needed to talk herself into driving at all. (Denise worked through this, with my help, and has stopped worrying about driving. It's totally possible to fix this without drugs or therapy.)

There's one last thing about the cortisol driving the reaction. Sometimes the cortisol is so high, so close to the physical state of anxiety, it really doesn't take anything to trigger the reaction. So we get anxious about, well, nothing.

Depression.

When I first read about depression and menopause, psychologists were still leaning toward the old Freudian models of human sexuality and behavior. Women became depressed at menopause because they were mourning the loss of fertility and were unhappy at getting older. For some women, that may be true. It's not the whole story, though, nor even correct in many cases.

True, there can be a sense of loss and a fear of getting old, much of which stems from our culture's obsession with youth and beauty. But depression actually has more to do with the hormonal changes than with these (or any) psychological factors.

From a physiological view, depression is linked to a lack of serotonin. For women, estrogen is a necessary ingredient in the synthesis of serotonin in the brain. When not enough estrogen is available, serotonin production suffers.

It happened to me. In my mid-forties, I started a downward spiral into depression. I was still very much in the early stages of perimenopause, which means I really didn't know what was happening to me. I wound up seeking help from a therapist, where a few weeks of traditional talk therapy convinced me I was fine. In truth, it was probably just another turn of the hormonal screw back to a temporarily more balanced state, because eventually, depression became my number one symptom. It wasn't until I started fixing my hormonal imbalances that depression stopped being a problem.

Mood swings.

Mood swings are a stereotypical symptom of menopause. In an iconic episode of "*All in the Family*" from 1972, "Edith's Problem," Jean Stapleton portrays Edith's entrance into menopause brilliantly (the episode is available on YouTube). On every entrance to the living room, she's in a different mood. Angry, happy, fearful, weepy. Your experience may be similar, or you may find your wife's moods change a little more slowly.

Mood swings are a result of fluctuating hormones and the neurotransmitters they influence. We tend to think of them as going from one negative emotion to another, but as the episode mentioned above shows, normal or happy emotions are thrown into the mix, too. The emotions that stand out, both to you and your wife, are the negative ones, though. That's because it may be abnormal for her to be expressing such strong negative emotions. Many women don't express their negative feelings in such definitive terms, but one of the results of lowered levels of estrogen is that women's "people pleasing" tendencies are also diminished.

While the emotions feel "over the top," the emotions underneath may be more authentic than she'll admit when the hormones aren't pushing the reaction.

Frustration and irritability.

While frustration and irritability are often part of the "mood swings," I think it's important to touch on emotional outbursts (or permanent states) of these two emotions in particular.

These two may be actual emotional reactions to what she's experiencing.

Imagine yourself in her place.

You've been going along knowing your body, knowing your cycle, understanding how you fit into your world. Then, along comes menopause. You never know when you're going to have a period. You don't know how you're going to feel. You can't predict anything, and you don't feel like yourself at all.

You react differently to things you've known all your life. You forget things, and you feel disorganized and incompetent.

You feel old, overnight.

Frustration and irritability can be reactions to her feeling out of place and unable to cope in her world. Wouldn't you feel that way?

Jesse says: I guess I'd being going crazy, too, if it were happening to me.

JEANNE D. ANDRUS
JESSE M. ANDRUS

Chapter 5
Her Changing Self

Your wife has been a great wife and mother. She's been a great employee. You're proud of the person she's been for all the years. Whether you were high school sweethearts or you're both on your second marriages or anything in between, you know her. She's always considerate and accommodating to everyone. She goes the extra mile. She takes care of everyone.

Or, at least she did.

Lately, she's been distant and self-involved. Or snappy and peevish. Or introverted and withdrawn.

You realize that her body is changing, but why does it seem that she isn't even the same person anymore? Where is your delightful social butterfly? The woman who could organize a class party while managing an important project at work and never miss a beat? What happened to decorations for every season, parties for every occasion, and nary a hair out of place?

The changes are more than just physical, emotional, and in the way she thinks.

The changes in her hormonal systems reverberate throughout her whole being. They can shake her to her core, calling into question her identity, her personal goals and vision for herself, and even her personality. Let me explain how that happens.

Her Changing Identity

When girls reach puberty, as defined by their first period, someone (usually their mother) is likely to tell her, "Now you are a woman." Her teen magazines (and especially the advertisers) tell her that her period defines her womanhood.

As she reaches the end of her high school and college years, she's told by our culture that her fertility defines her. Yes, this comes through even as we've opened up opportunities for careers for women and made non-traditional paths more acceptable. But the subtext is still there.

In the book, *Flow* (Stein & Kim, 2009), our worth is described this way: "On a planet where for thousands of years, even today, a woman's worth has been judged exclusively by the productivity of her womb, what the h**l is the point of a barren woman?" Wow! That pretty much summarizes what we've been told by society all our lives.

Then, our periods stop. We can no longer bear children. It doesn't matter whether we've had no children or a houseful. We've lost our identity as women.

And we're wondering. Who are we? *What* are we?

A change that big takes some getting used to. It's not that we are looking to get pregnant now (although sometimes our body suggests we might like to have another baby, mostly our rational mind screams, "Nooooo!"). But all our adult lives, our identity has been tied up with the notion that we *might* get pregnant.

Just as important, our lives have been dictated by a certain physical rhythm, as we have lived with the monthly cycle of our periods. Whether we experience the larger emotional and physical shifts of premenstrual syndrome (PMS) or not, we are used to the changes in our emotions and bodies and sexuality that governs our lives. Ask any woman where she is in her cycle and, even if she isn't thinking about it, she can check in with her body and tell you how close her period is.

Now, menopause changes all that. Our cycles are shorter or longer. We skip periods or have periods that last seemingly forever. There's no predictability. The other parts of us, like our emotions and our sexuality and even our thinking, are shifting around. We can't count on ourselves to be the person we expect to be.

Oh, and one more thing. No one tells us this is going to happen, and the most iconic role models we have for this stage of our lives are the witches, hags, and evil stepmothers of the fairy tales of our youth.

Is it any wonder that we're kinda confused by the whole thing?

Her Changing Goals and Personal Vision

Once she realizes that she's not the same person she was, whether it's conscious or sub-conscious, she may start re-evaluating who she wants to be for the rest of her life. That's actually one of the best things about menopause, but it can be very disconcerting for a woman and for the people in her life.

She's also concerned about "getting old." For most of human history, the majority of women didn't reach menopause, and those who did had only a short life expectancy left. We're conditioned to think of menopause as coming at the end of life. It doesn't help that some of the side effects of diminishing estrogen include some of the changes that are typically identified with aging (like wrinkles, thinning skin, graying hair, achy joints, and more).

I know that when I thought about myself as old (I wasn't even close to being old, I know now), I started thinking about what I hadn't yet done in my life. It was more than crossing items off a bucket list. I hadn't yet achieved what I wanted to in my life.

For me, there was the realization that the goals I'd been pursuing weren't fulfilling. Yes, I'd raised a great kid and had an interesting career. I'd mentored younger team members and made a difference to the projects I was on. It wasn't enough. I wanted more.

This may happen to your partner, as well. She may sit down with herself and realize that she's missed out on the most important things she'd like to accomplish. Those could be career goals – things like starting a business, or going in a different direction. It could be personal goals, like traveling or competing in a specific arena. It could be associated with volunteering or writing or living on a farm or just about anything.

Whatever it is, it will be important to her. And she'll want to achieve it.

Her Changing Personality

One of the odd things about menopause is that for some women, it changes some aspects of their personality. Well, I shouldn't say it quite like that. Because what happens is that estrogen has altered her personality for most of her adult life. It's made her more willing to work cooperatively and be part of a community effort. It may have made her more extroverted. It may have made her more verbal.

When estrogen recedes, she may become more herself than ever before. And that may be a person you've never actually met. And that opens up a world of opportunities for an even better relationship than before.

What Does It All Mean?

You may have been your wife's partner for many, many years, or you may have only recently met and married. Whichever it is, your relationship was most likely based on the person your wife has been up until now – up until her menopausal journey started.

Now, she's changing. She can't help it. Her body is driving the changes and the changes are pre-programmed. They are her destiny at this time of her life. And they aren't particularly easy changes.

She may have some information or not much information at all. If she hasn't already, I really recommend she read my first book, *I Just Want to Be ME Again!* I designed it as a primer of the information a woman really needs to survive and thrive during menopause, and while the information in this book is accurate, it's still just the "owner's manual." She needs the Chilton's manual to her body.

She may be scared or just plain angry at the changes she's going through. She could be confused.

She might be excited about the possibilities opening up for her, or depressed about the doors closing behind her.

Whatever she's feeling, it's a pretty safe bet that she's hoping that you'll provide the right kind of support for her now.

JEANNE D. ANDRUS
JESSE M. ANDRUS

Chapter 6
Her Changing Libido

Have you been noticing a certain chilliness lately? For many men, what happens now in the bedroom is both a literal and a metaphorical chill. And I want to address both.

Jesse says: I did notice it was getting cool at night, and I don't just mean because I'm wearing a sweatshirt to bed.

Night Sweats

So, let's talk about the literal chilliness of your bedroom first, because that's actually a bit easier to deal with than the chill between you and her.

Night sweats. They're the nighttime version of hot flashes and they're about 20 times more annoying. It's estimated that hot flashes and night sweats affect up to three-quarters of all women going through menopause.

Night sweats can happen a couple of different ways.

For one woman, it's like being that proverbial frog in a pot of cold water. She gets into bed, and sometimes she's even cold, so she snuggles down into the covers like she's been doing for the last 40 or so years. She falls asleep, all curled up in a nest. And, because she's a little chilly, her body starts to warm up. The heat doesn't escape because she's under the duvet. And her internal thermostat never shuts down. She keeps heating up and the heat doesn't escape, until she feels like she just burst into flames.

For another, it's a flush that begins in her chest area and zooms up her neck and engulfs her whole head. Her scalp is perspiring and her upper body is drenched in sweat. For her, her feet could still be cold, but putting them under the blankets just results in more heat in her chest, neck, and head.

Either way, she can soak a pair of pajamas and the sheets in no time at all. She's wide awake, and she feels like her hair is on fire. If you feel the pillow where her head was, it's almost too hot to touch.

If she's not prepared for it, now she's wide awake. The room feels like the fires of Hades are reaching in and toasting her like a marshmallow over a campfire. She's soaked, and there may be nothing clean and dry to put on.

Now, in her damp nightgown, she wanders into the bathroom, taking a drink of water to cool down and to try and regroup. She glances at the clock. One o'clock. There's a lot of night left. And then the bottom falls out, and she's cold. The damp of her gown chills her. She returns to the bed, and tosses and turns: sometimes too hot, sometimes too cold. Another night with lousy sleep.

That's why the thermostat in your room is set to 3 degrees below freezing, and she still curses the heat. Everyone's body comes with a great temperature regulation system, unless you're a woman and have reached menopause. Then, it malfunctions, and you never know when it's going to happen.

No one's really sure why women have hot flashes. For some women, they seem to happen due to minute-to-minute fluctuations in hormones and for others, they seem to be related to low estrogen. Still others seem related to an imbalance between progesterone and estrogen. But whatever causes them, they are hard to take and almost impossible to control.

Jesse says: However you like the bedroom - hot or cold - it really

doesn't matter. She's going to win this one. You can put on a sweatshirt (like me), or buy an electric blanket, or even sleep in another room. It's just not worth fighting over. The better she sleeps, the better my wife treats me!

The "Other" Chill

Then there's that other chill you may be feeling. Has it been too long since she reached for you, or even didn't reject your advances when you reached for her?

Sex becomes a distant memory for way too many couples in mid-life. And that can put a strain on your relationship. She says she loves you, but she rejects you in the bedroom. Or she's distant. Or you don't get any feedback at all – she just lies there. Or worse yet, you realize it hurts for her. I know you don't want that.

Before we get in to fixing the problem (in Part Two), let's talk about some of the things that are happening that are getting in the way.

Physical changes.
There are two changes in her hormones that are affecting her physical response to sex. The first is a drop in estrogen that can cause changes in her vaginal tissues that make sex uncomfortable. Vaginal dryness and vaginal atrophy affect many women, especially once their periods are done (or when there's a gap of several months between periods).

When sex becomes uncomfortable or even painful, it's pretty certain that she's not going to respond positively to your advances or initiate any on her own. It also means that a certain amount of preparation and adjustment will be necessary in order for her to not be in pain during sex.

The second issue is decreasing testosterone. Yes, she has testosterone, too. For her, testosterone means a few things. First, it helps her build and retain muscle. Second, it helps her feel motivated and assertive. And finally, it has a close tie to her sex drive.

Testosterone naturally drops in everyone after the age of 40. For some women, this drop can be enough that their sex drive and ability to be aroused becomes almost non-existent. In most cases, this means that she'd like to be in the mood for sex, but when the moment comes, in the words of one of my clients, "nothing's going on down there."

Emotional changes.

More significantly, she is changing emotionally, and that affects how she responds to sex. There are many potential conflicts, so I want to discuss just a few of them. In Part Two, we'll talk about how to approach the subject with your wife so you can understand what's going on with her, in particular. (Until then, please refrain from playing amateur psychologist – that can do more harm than good.)

She's bone tired. I'm leading off with this one, because I think that we neglect how important the role of good rest is in helping women feel interested in sex (and in anything other than finally getting a good night's sleep).

Remember that thing about hot flashes disturbing her sleep? The truth of the matter is that the hormonal changes of menopause can disturb her sleep in numerous ways. And she's still got work and the house and the kids to deal with. She's tired. And sex is just one more chore on her list. No wonder she's not terribly enthusiastic.

She thinks you can't possibly want sex with her. Most of us see the physical changes of menopause – weight shift and gain, hairs where they've never been before, wrinkles, and more – as signs of aging. And, of course, our culture revolves around youth as beauty. So, what does that make us? Old, fat, and ugly. Our bodies have betrayed us. You can't possibly be interested in sex with us. When you run your hand over our belly fat, we're reminded of it, and we recoil from the body we now hate.

Jesse says: I will always see my wife as beautiful, because she's the woman I love.

Most women don't realize that you don't care about any of that. You have been with her through thick and thin, and you still love her. And you want to express that physically.

She wants a different relationship with you. In Chapter Nine, we're going to talk about renegotiating your relationship – why the two of you might need to redefine your life together. Sex might very well be part of that. She may want or need a different type of sexual relationship. She may need more stimulation or more romance or more cuddling. She may need more date nights, or more conversation.

As a part of examining and rebuilding your relationship, take the time to talk through your sex life. What are your desires? What would be perfection in your mind? Then, what are hers? What would she like to have happen in the bedroom?

Remember, too, that women are much more emotionally and mentally involved in sex than men. For most men, sex is mostly a physical thing. For most women, sex is something that happens inside a committed and emotional relationship. If your relationship is strained or distant, if you two have become more like roommates than lovers, you may have to work first at the relationship in order for sex to become more appealing to her.

She expects her sex drive to go down. I know this sounds weird, but many women talk with each other about how they're just not interested anymore. If that's what she's hearing, and you're not taking the time to romance her and engage her before you initiate sex, she may be feeling that she shouldn't be interested anymore.

She's redefining herself. As she moves from being a mother, both in actuality and in the way she perceives herself, she may be looking to expand her life in ways that don't involve sex. After estrogen begins to drop, she may find herself looking at the things that she may have given up for raising a family, being a wife and mother, and maybe building a "career" that wasn't quite what she thought it would be.

One of the reactions to menopause I've seen over and over is that women want "more" – we want to be what we might have been, or to embrace a dream that we've found along to the way. Maybe it's to travel around the world, or work with animals, or write, or be an artist. But that passion reawakens in us.

So, what does that have to do with sex? Sometimes, it's that she becomes wrapped up in that passion and forgets to make room in her life for what's been there all along. Or, it could be that she sees you as part of the old life. She doesn't know how to fit you into the new life she's building.

What Do You Do About Sex?

In Part Two, I'd like to talk about how you and your partner can deal with the change that is menopause as a couple. If you're like my husband, you're going to want to "cut to the chase" and skip right to the chapter on how you can make your sex life better.

I'm going to suggest that you don't do that. The way you'll get to a better sex life is to support your wife as she goes through menopause. Part Two is all about how you support her. The techniques I'll be recommending may not be the same as the ones you've used to deal with problems in your life and your relationship. If they were, I wouldn't have needed to write Part Two. In fact, I probably wouldn't have had to write this book at all.

So, indulge me. Read all of Part Two. If you think I'm describing something that you don't need to do in your relationship, ask your wife. If she agrees with you, you can skip it. But, I bet she won't. I bet she'll be surprised and pleased by your consideration of her feelings.

JEANNE D. ANDRUS
44 JESSE M. ANDRUS

Part Two:
You Can't Fix This with a Pipe Wrench

I remember after my son was grown and on his own, we were walking and talking on one of his rare visits home. I was probably frustrated with something at my job and taking advantage of his presence to complain about it.

I wasn't looking for answers; I just needed someone to listen for a bit and help me feel vindicated. I wanted to know that someone was on my side, ready to ride into battle for me, should I need it. I didn't need it and, of course, it would have been wildly inappropriate for my 25-year-old son to go to my place of employment and tell them to stop picking on his mom.

At one point, after I'd rejected his fifth or sixth suggestion for ways to handle the situation, he stopped me. He said, "You don't really *want* my help on this, do you?"

"Not particularly," I replied. "But there's not a lot of people around I can say this to, and you're handy."

"Oh," he said. "I thought when people talked about a problem, they wanted a solution."

"Not always," I answered. "Especially women. Sometimes, we just want to talk about it and feel like someone's listening."

He thought about that for a moment and said, "But guys don't feel comfortable unless they're fixing things."

If you're a "fixer," like my son, menopause is going to stymie and frustrate you.

First and most important, the fixes aren't necessarily easy, and your wife has got to make the changes herself. Because many of the symptoms aren't even easily detected from outside (they have to do with the way she feels, both emotionally and in her body), you won't know exactly what she's trying to fix and she might not know how to describe what's going on.

Second, many of the best ways to affect the symptoms positively are changes to diet, as well as exercise and stress management. And if you've been through diets with your wife before, you already know that spouses are not usually the best diet coaches, accountability partners, and peers. Men and women diet differently, exercise differently, and even de-stress differently. Unless you've done this stuff together often, you probably don't want to be the one to ask her if she really wants that doughnut. Especially if the thirty-third day of a non-stop period already has her in a pretty bad mood.

The third problem with your role as a handyman is that I've noticed (and I may be way off base here, but just consider it) that fixers tend to want to fix other people's problems. As you go through this section, notice that a lot of what's happening is that you and your wife are rebuilding your relationship with yourselves and with each other. That means that you're going to need to make some changes and fixes to yourself as well.

Finally, I'm going to caution you, before we get going, about Googling "what to do for your wife in menopause" and reading and following articles that don't get any deeper than advice like "give her a foot rub, always put her car keys back on their hook when you find them in the refrigerator, and buy her flowers." There's something to be said for foot rubs, but these suggestions are just the tip of the iceberg.

So let's get started.

JEANNE D. ANDRUS
JESSE M. ANDRUS

Chapter 7

Here It Is:
How to Reignite Your Sex Life with Your Wife

I know you've been waiting for this chapter, so let's get right to it....

It's not about sex. Not this chapter, anyway.

Jesse says: What? You tricked me. I looked here first.

Now, before you go looking for the real chapter about sex, there's a reason I want you reading this chapter now! Because it's really more important to read this and the next couple of chapters if you want to have a wonderful, full life with your wife, including a great sex life.

Here's why. You've heard it before – men make love with their bodies, women make love with their hearts and minds. And right now, your wife's mind and heart may not be that into sex (and her body probably isn't, either). So, for the next several chapters, I going to share with you my best advice about how to help your wife through menopause. Because that's how you're going to have your best relationship, in every way, with your wife.

So, stick with me here. And I promise we'll get back to what happens in the bedroom.

Then what are we going to talk about in this chapter? We're going to talk about what not to do.

Don't: Take It Personally

Just like your wife probably does some things you don't like, you probably do some things she doesn't like. That's pretty much human nature. None of us likes every choice and every action and every word of anyone else. Even the person we love with all our heart.

For the first few decades of her life, your wife was designed to let those things go (she might not have done so, but her hormones were saying, "Make peace. It's no big deal."). Now, she's changing and things that might merely have been annoying a few years ago are now big issues, and she's wondering why you continue to do something that you know drives her crazy.

"What? What? What did I do?" is your response.

"You know I hate it when you do that." she says in response.

"That? I didn't know you didn't like it when I [fill in the blank]."

"Yes, you do. You remember. I told you the weekend Ellen [your daughter] had her friend, Joan, over and we cooked barbeque."

You, of course, barely remember your own daughter's name, much less her friend, Joan, and you sure don't remember that cookout or the discussion. But she does.

I'm sure you're ready to explode. Of course you are. It's not fair of her to expect you to remember that. But if you explode, she'll explode back and there will be a fight.

Instead, don't take it personally. It's the difference in the way her brain works and the way yours does. She remembers those kinds of interpersonal interactions; you remember how to fix a carburetor. If you want to go for extra credit, apologize for not remembering the conversation and for continuing to do something that's annoying to her.

Don't: Explain Her Body to Her

When I set out to write this book, I actually worried about including the informational sections for you. I worried about telling you what was going on in her body and how it affects her. Because one thing that men do that drives most women, especially their wives, crazy is to explain to them the things they already know. And, it might be a temptation for you to explain it to her.

So I tried to make sure you'd read this chapter first. (Hence the sneaky title.)

You might be tempted to Google her symptoms, or the topic of menopause. You might want to go to her gynecologist with her. I'm going to suggest you don't do any of that. Not without asking her what she wants from you.

Worst of all, you might want to "diagnose" her, saying something like, "I know your moodiness is due to your lack of estrogen, since you're perimenopausal." A jury of her peers (i.e., menopausal women) would never convict her on the charges the district attorney would probably want to bring. Justifiable homicide would be the verdict.

It is true that she might not know everything she needs to know about the changes her body is going through. It may even be true that she is unaware of how she appears to other people (depressed or angry or moody).

Your role, though, is to be supportive where she needs it. And, while we're at it, that brings up another "don't."

Don't: Take Over Her Menopause

What do I mean by that?

Let's look at what's happened around another physical change of women's bodies – pregnancy. When I was a child, when a couple started expecting a child, she was pregnant. Men would say, "My wife's expecting." Sure, they'd burst with pride from their part in it, but they weren't pregnant. Now, it's the *couple* that's pregnant. "We're pregnant!" he announces to his buddies, "We're having a baby!" Technically – no. She's pregnant. She's getting the morning sickness, gaining the weight, and she can't even have a glass of wine. She's in labor; she gets to push, and she's going through the childbirth. But she won't tell you that, because she wants you as involved as possible.

Menopause is hers. She gets to be the star (whether she wants to or not), and she gets to go through it the way she wants. Let her have it; don't try to be the expert or take credit for it.

You're the supporting actor in this piece. You get to follow her lead. Trust me, this is a great place not to be in the leading role!

Jesse says: I definitely don't to be the star of this one.

Don't: Be Her Coach or Her Accountability Partner

Whenever one of my clients decides to make changes in her lifestyle, especially around diet, exercise, or smoking, we talk about the role their spouse will play in helping them make the changes. Invariably, their reaction to their spouse as their accountability partner is "Oh, h**l no!" The thoughts of their spouse telling them what or when they can eat or telling them to go workout, set their teeth on edge.

Here's the thing. Your wife is an adult, and more than ever before, she sees herself as an equal partner in your relationship. She doesn't want you bossing her around. She wants to be able to make her own decisions, even if it's a decision she might regret later.

Yes, you'll have a role in whatever she decides. You may be a workout partner or you may help her get the right foods at the grocery store. Or you might decide you need to make some lifestyle changes yourself and ask her to help you. Together, you might agree that certain reminders are okay and others are off-limits.

We'll talk more about these types of negotiations in the next couple of chapters. Right now, just remember you aren't Mickey Goldmill getting Rocky in shape for the fight. You're an occasional training partner. If she decides she's going to sleep in and skip her morning workout, it's not your job to make her feel guilty.

Don't: Try to Fix Things

I've already said it. You just can't fix this. Maybe some small things, but not the big thing. You can't make menopause go away or go any faster or really change her experience from a physical sense.

What she wants you to do is listen. She wants someone to be on her side. She wouldn't complain if you brought her flowers or rubbed her feet. She might want someone to be outraged at the doctor or her boss or the clerk who offered her a "senior citizen discount." But she wouldn't be happy if you hopped in the car and drove to the store and yelled at the clerk.

If That's What Not to Do, What Do You Do?

Jesse says: That list of "don'ts" is all the things you thought you could do for her, isn't it? When she told me that, I said, "So what the heck

am I supposed to do? Just let you be miserable?" And then she told me. Maybe I should have just let her be miserable. No, just kidding.

In our next two chapters, I'll tell you what I told Jesse and how we got through my menopause. We're going to look at the things you can do to support your wife and strengthen your relationship.

Chapter 8
It's Time We Had a T.A.L.K.

I'm going to admit that I have no idea what your wife really needs from you as she goes through menopause.

But, don't throw this book away just yet! I know, I know. You're probably thinking why the heck did you even start reading this book if I wasn't going to tell you what to do. But I **am** going to tell you what to do. Exactly what to do.

I don't know what her needs are. Her needs and wants are just as unique and personal as she is. They'll change as she goes through her menopausal journey. So, if I tried to give you a few actions to take, I'd probably fail miserably. I'd rather show you a method for finding out what she needs and wants at any given time.

The method is fairly easy. It's just T.A.L.K. Sitting down and talking. But it's more than that. It's a specific sequence of communicating in ways designed to elicit her needs and help her understand that you will do your best to make things better for her.

In this case, T.A.L.K. stands for Tell, Ask, Listen, and K(c)ommit. You'll *tell* her that you are concerned and interested. You'll *ask* her how you can support her. You'll *listen* (with active listening skills) to her response. Finally, you'll know what actions you'll be taking, and she'll know what *commitment* you've made.

The T.A.L.K. Method

Let's examine this method a little more deeply.

Tell – Tell her you're interested and ready to support her

The first step is to let your wife know that you realize that menopause is probably creating havoc in her life. This isn't a litany of the symptoms you've noticed, but simply a recognition that you've found out enough about the process that you're aware that this isn't an easy process. (If she gave you this book, it's probably easier to broach the subject!)

There's something else you need to tell her. You need to tell her that you care about her and that you're in it for the long haul. She's likely not feeling really great about herself. She needs to hear that you care about her.

More than that, she needs to believe it. I know you mean it. I know you think it should be enough to just say it. But believe me, she's lost her confidence. She's unsure of herself. She doesn't know why you'd want to stick around or what you see in her. She's afraid that you're going to walk away, and she's afraid that she doesn't know how to keep you.

If you're not sure how to convince her that you're in this with her, I often recommend that my clients and their spouses look at how they express love to one another. An easy way to do this is to use the framework developed by Gary Chapman called *"The Five Love Languages."* (Chapman has made a whole franchise out of this concept, but you may not need more than this brief introduction.)

The five "languages" are ways we give and receive love. Even if you or your wife use a language that doesn't fall into one of the five, you can look at how you express love and how she receives it. One suggestion I make for my clients is to use all five (or more, if you have them) love languages to express your feelings to your spouse. Right now, she's feeling especially vulnerable, and she needs a lot of reassurance.

Language One – Words. Obviously, the words you say, and the words you don't say, are part of your expression of love. Say the good ones, save the jokes, the subtle insults, or the put-downs for a few years (or forever).

Language Two – Physical Touching. Little touches, quick kisses, a hug here and there goes a long way to saying, "I love you and care about you." So do shoulder rubs, scalp massages, and just general pampering. But they don't replace saying the words.

Language Three – Small Gifts. Bringing home a small treat, flowers or a special chocolate, a pair of earrings – these are a great ways to say, "I care." Bigger gifts are wonderful, but it's the little things that say you're thinking of her when you're out and about. Just make it something that's chosen for her. Some women like flowers, others would prefer a plant for their garden.

Language Four – Acts of Kindness. The little things that you can do that make her life easier or better. Wash or vacuum her car (or take it to the car wash). Stop to pick up the groceries or the dry cleaning. Set up that appointment, and get the dog to the vet. I'm not talking about doing your share of the chores. This love language means that you are taking some of her work away from her.

Language Five – Quality Time. Sometimes, all it takes to say, "I love you," is to spend time with each other. The key is that you're doing something she wants to do. It could be going to the movie she wants to see or doing a jigsaw puzzle together or playing tennis. Sometimes, you complete a chore or an errand together. Other times, it's just decompressing at the end of the day together.

Choose your languages and express your caring and love frequently. The voices in her head have her questioning her own beauty and worth and it may take more for her to believe in herself as the symptoms and changes of menopause take over her thinking.

Jesse says: This is not a "one-and-done" kinda thing. And it's worth it. Because the more you do for her, the more she'll return back to you.

Ask – Let her tell you what she needs or wants from you

Jesse says: No, "A" doesn't stand for assume! She's pounded that into my brain way too often. Yes, I'm the ass in "making an ass-umption." I don't assume anymore.

Asking questions is the way you're going to figure out what she needs from you.

When you first start asking, you may not get a good answer. She might not be used to expressing her needs this way. She might not know what she needs. She might be embarrassed at what she needs or explaining her symptoms.

I'm asking you not to take the easy way out. It's simple to say, "Okay. I asked. She said she didn't need anything from me. We're good." The truth is, though, she needs more than that. She needs you to keep asking. She needs you to ask in different words and different ways. All without bugging her. (I know, we're not really rational. That's just the way it is.)

A couple of tips for probing for what she needs:

- Ask open ended questions. Questions that can be answered yes or no shut down conversation. Ask questions that need a sentence (or an essay) to answer. A question like "Can I do anything for you?" results in a quick "No." Asking "How can I help you today?" is better. Even better "Tell me what you're feeling about the changes, please."

- Ask for more. "Tell me more about [whatever she just told you]" is a conversation-starter. Just agreeing with her shuts conversation down, even if she thinks that's a good thing.

That brings us to the "L" in TALK – Listen.

Listen – **Paying attention to her experience**

So often, we listen in order to formulate our response to what's being said. We all do it. Every one of us. When we think have enough to respond, usually with a great response that proves we know oh, so much about the topic at hand, we stop listening and work on improving our response.

The problem with that approach? We miss so much of what's said. We probably miss the most important parts of what we're being told.

But when we listen deeply to what's being said to us, it's definitely worthwhile. First, there's a lot more information forthcoming. And you get the clues that allow you to probe more deeply (Ask more). Most importantly, there's the improved relationship from being the person who listens and hears. Because none of us feels listened to enough. And your wife will love being heard.

Here are some "active listening" techniques that help you to really hear what's being said to you.

Don't interrupt. Use body language and facial expressions as you listen to show that you're hearing what's being said. Let her speak until she's done and ask a "tell me more" type question to elicit anything else she is feeling. Make it clear that you are paying attention.

Reflective listening. In reflective listening, you state back what you've heard in order to verify that you heard correctly. In most cases, you want to change the words, so she doesn't feel like she's talking to a parrot. There are two types of reflective listening. In simple reflective listening, you restate what you've heard. There's also complex reflective listening, in which you take a stab at the underlying meaning. If you do that, always phrase it as a question, so that your wife can confirm your inquiry or guide you further.

Summarizing. Summarizing is a technique of restating a longer thought into a shorter framing of it. Just as with reflective listening, allow for the possibility that you've heard it wrong. If so, don't take it personally. Listen to the feedback and keep reflecting, restating, and summarizing until she agrees that you understand her point of view.

Don't try to fix the problem. (Yeah, I said it again.) While your spouse may give you specific things that she'd like you to do to help her, it's not up to you to provide solutions. Not trying to fix the problem gives you the freedom to hear what she is saying and to allow and assist her to come up with her own solutions.

Kommit (okay, it really starts with a C, but it should start with a K) – Promise your help the way she wants it

Jesse says: Women! They care about spelling, until they want to misspell something!

Once she's identified the problem and the way she wants you to help her, then your job is to promise that support. It may even be that she wants you to do some of the things I suggested that you don't do. That's okay. If she asks you to help in that way, it's because that's what she needs.

I'm going to guess, though, that many of the ways she'll want your support will be things like:

- "Understand that I don't always have control over the way I react." The women I coach are often looking for feeling better and having more control over their emotions and bodies. And, for the most part, they achieve that. But, not always. And when that happens, your understanding will go a long way to making it easier on her.

- "Cut me some slack around the house." She may have symptoms that are making her tired or sore, and it's hard to get things done. She may just not care as much about how the house looks and whether the chores are done. She wants your "permission" to not be perfect in this realm.

- "Keep telling me you love me, even though I'm not young and beautiful anymore." Her symptoms often make her question whether she's worthy of your love. They can disrupt her libido and even her ability to have sex. She's scared you're going to trade her for a "newer model."

Once you commit, carry through. If you choose to support her now, the relationship you have now will sustain you both for decades to come.

JEANNE D. ANDRUS
JESSE M. ANDRUS

Chapter 9
Recreate Your Relationship

Your wife is going through a period of big physical changes. That's a given with menopause.

But, chances are there are lots of other changes coming up in your lives, because you're at the age when those changes tend to occur.

If your family is like many of the families of the women I work with, here are just some of the changes you may be facing or contemplating:

- Your children are beginning to become independent adults, leaving for college or even graduating and beginning their own lives.

- Your parents may be declining and considering late life options (such as assisted living or moving to retirement homes, or even hospice). You and your wife may be finding yourself in the role of caregivers or decision-makers for incapacitated parents. You may even be facing losing them.

- Careers may be stalled or ending, as you and/or your wife find that they are no longer fulfilling, financially as well as emotionally/mentally.

- Retirement may be on the horizon, with financial considerations and the desire to realize long-postponed dreams, hopes, and plans (moving to new locations, traveling, building a business around a passion, volunteering for a cause long important to you).

- Health considerations, including concerns surrounding genetic predispositions toward disabling conditions.

- Financially, you may not be in the position you had hoped to be by this time, making decisions about all of the above issues more stressful.

And in the midst of all this, you are both going through physical changes that alter how you perceive and relate to the world. Menopause for her and andropause for you. (If you don't know about your changing body and what andropause is and how it affects you, check the "further resources" page for some places to get more information.)

All of that adds up to stress. Lots of stress.

Is it any wonder then, that the relationship you two may have begun when you were in your twenties seems like it's not quite the same?

That doesn't mean that you need just cut your losses and walk away.

I assume that the reason you're reading this book is because you want to improve this relationship you've nurtured for many years. I hope that your love for your wife is still intact, and you'd like to keep this marriage going for years to come. I'm guessing that every time you see a picture of some adorable old couple celebrating their 60th anniversary, you imagine yourself and your wife as that couple.

How are you going to do that?

Get to Know Each Other Again

There's a very strong likelihood that you and your wife are different people than the people you were when you married. Since then, you've made a home together, maybe had kids and raised them, perhaps gone through a career change or two. Certainly, the world around you has changed. Economic changes, political changes, social changes, technological changes. I spent years working in a career that wasn't invented when I went to college and I have hobbies now that weren't invented then, either.

It's really common that we don't grow and change in lockstep with our partners. I'm sure that you still share many interests and, of course, you've got zillions of memories that you've made together. But that doesn't mean you still know each other the way you did when you were "courting."

Do you know your best friend and soulmate the way that you did back then?

Or do you know the wife and mother she's been for the last 20 or 30 years?

It's time to get to know the woman you're married to. What's changed in her way of thinking and feeling? What are the important life lessons she's learned as she's gone through life? What are the dreams and hopes she has for the future?

Remember how we outlined the "TALK" method of communicating in the last chapter? It's time to bring it out and put it to practice in finding out all about this "new" woman in your life.

Don't know where to start? How about starting with a great set of questions?

In 1997, psychologist Arthur Aron published a study about the development of intimacy. He developed a set of 36 questions that he felt would lead to intimacy between two people who seriously answered them with each other. This list became wildly popular again in this decade and was the subject of numerous magazine articles and even an episode of the TV program *The Big Bang Theory*.

You may think you could answer these questions for your partner, but if you actually commit to the exercise, you may learn that she's changed in some surprising ways.

You can find a list of these questions here (http://bigthink.com/ideafeed/how-to-fall-in-love-36-questions-and-deep-eye-contact). You'll notice they are divided into three sets. After completing the questions, the directions suggest you gaze into each other's eyes for three to four minutes.

Jesse says: You mean, like a staring contest?

No, Jess. Just gaze into each other's eyes.

Given your level of relationship, you might do one set of questions (and eye contact) on each of three "date nights." Make sure you have a quiet space to talk, and take turns answering each question. Feel free to add questions about your own situation and future.

Change Yourself First

Are there things wrong with her? Of course there are! She's not perfect. There are plenty of things she should change. Even she'd admit that (but maybe not to you).

But here's the thing. You can't change her.

No one can change anyone else. Not true, deep change.

The only person you have a chance of changing is yourself. And you have to want to do it.

Jesse says: Q: How many psychologists does it take to change a lightbulb? A: Only one, but the lightbulb has to really want to change.

One way to change is start with thinking about who the person is who can contribute positively to your relationship. Here are some questions you can start with to define who you want to be in this relationship:

- What do you want to accomplish in the rest of your life? (See, it's not all about her. Your needs count, too.)

- What do you want more of in your life?

- What things in your life aren't serving you anymore (things, relationships, habits, activities)? Should you let them go?

- What have you let go that you shouldn't have? Can you bring them back (or bring them back in a new way)?

- What do you want your relationship with your wife to be?

Now, how can you take one step today toward becoming the person you want to be? Each day, ask yourself this question and take that one step. It could be little or it could be big, but if you take that step, you'll be one step closer to being the best you ever. The you you'd like to be.

You Can't "Help Around the House"

When I was a new mom, a guy I worked with mentioned that he had to get home to "babysit." I nearly lost it. "You can't babysit your own kids," I told him. He was confused by the concept. I explained that babysitting was something that a relative stranger did either as a favor or for pay. Parents take care of their kids. Either together or individually. Childcare isn't "her job" that you "helped with" occasionally. It's a joint responsibility.

Household chores are the same thing. Especially now that your lives are changing.

You may have grown up in a household with a stay-at-home mom. The house and the kids were her domain, and she took care of everything involved with that domain. She cleaned the house, and cooked and cleaned up afterwards. She decorated for holidays and shopped for everyone's gifts. She was the "room mother" at your school and the den mother for your cub scout pack.

Your dad may have had his "honey do" list for the weekends, but that revolved around "manly" chores – mowing the lawn, repairing the washing machine, replanting your mom's favorite rosebush. (Yes, I'm playing on stereotypes here. Most of us remember these stereotypes as real. Even though my mom worked outside the home, the "division of labor" was still very traditional in my house.)

As an adult, you may have realized that it wasn't completely fair that your wife worked a full-time job and then came home to a second job of keeping house and caring for the kids. You might have realized that you had equal responsibility to your children.

But when it came to the house, you probably thought of yourself as "helping around the house." The split of the chores could have been equitable, or she could have had the lion's share of the responsibility. Somehow, though, when you're "helping," it still feels like she's still carrying the whole load. In truth, often she is. She decides the menus even if you cook sometimes. She makes the chore list and divides it up, reminds you to take out the garbage, and she's the one who takes the morning off when the plumber gets called.

Now that your lives are changing, maybe it's time to change the way chores get divided up in your house. It may be time you took co-ownership of the job of keeping the house going. I do want to let you know that your wife may be perfectly happy with the way things are going, but it's up to you to verify that with her.

Jesse says: Does this mean that she'll mow the lawn and take out the garbage?
Not hardly, Jesse, not hardly. It's supposed to get easier for her.

Dream Together for the Future

You may have had a common goal that fueled your partnership when you first started out and were scrimping and saving to buy a house, or when you were raising your children. That kind of dedication to the same end probably brought you closer and kept your relationship on track.

Do you, as a couple, have a shared vision for your future?

Where do you want to be in the future as a family?

What is your dream come true as you move from raising a family to being "empty-nesters?"

Now, do you know with absolute, 100% certainty how your wife would answer those questions? Oh, and you'll only know with 100% certainty if you have talked to her about it recently. Because even if you know what it was, it may have changed.

If not, it's time to sit down and dream big together. Build a future in your imagination. See yourselves creating this future together. Examine how your relationship works in this future.

Are both of you getting everything you ever wanted? If not, can you tweak the dream so that you both are 100% fulfilled? How does that feel? (Yes, there may be places where one or both of you has to compromise – you can't live 100% of the time on the west coast and 100% of the time in Florida, but you can split your time 50/50.)

When you create a dream that both of you agree on, once again you have a common project to work toward. And you have a relationship with somewhere to go. Together.

Chapter 10
There Is Hope

Now that you and your partner have renegotiated your relationship and you've found the best way to support her through the changes that she's going through, let's talk about getting back to an active sex life. There are great reasons for both of you to maintain an active and satisfying sexual relationship.

Sex keeps the two of you close. It reinforces your relationship. If it's satisfying, it keeps both of you from injecting something or someone into your relationship that drives you apart.

Sex is good for your body. Sex is part of a healthy life, and it's been shown that those with an active sex life have better health and even live longer. It can release stress and enhance the levels of "feel good" hormones like serotonin, endorphins, and oxytocin (the cuddle hormone).

Sex is great for your brain. Studies have shown that those with an active sex life have a reduced risk of all forms of dementia.

So, how do you rebuild a healthy, active sex life?

Don't Take It Personally

Jesse says: I don't ever get to take anything personally, do I?

First and most importantly, the changes in your sex life are most likely not about you (especially if you've already worked through the suggestions in Chapter Nine). If she's dealing with a lowered libido due to hormonal changes, it wouldn't matter if you actually looked like that movie star she frequently remarks on. She would find herself uninterested in more than a platonic relationship with him in short order.

If she's dealing with physical changes that make sex painful (or even less pleasurable), it wouldn't matter who she was with. Sex would not be an option.

If she's discovered a new passion, whether it's art or travel or microbiology, she may just not have "looked up" from this new interest to see that your relationship needs nurturing.

Whatever the case, most likely, it's not you. It's just where she is now. Don't take it personally.

Jesse says: Yeah, well, I guess I don't want to take that personally.

Talk About It

The first piece of getting back to a passionate and fulfilling sex life is to talk about it. This is a discussion that needs to take place outside of the bedroom. It certainly shouldn't happen over a failed sexual encounter **(Jesse says: been there, done that – I hope never again!)**. There are a couple of important questions that the two of you need to answer together.

Do you have a relationship you both want to maintain?
Hopefully you didn't skip Chapter Nine and you've dealt with the essential questions about your relationship. If you did skip Chapter Nine, it's time to go back and rebuild your relationship. It's time to know that you both are fully invested in this relationship and want to move forward.

If not, if you aren't both fully committed to this relationship, what do you want to do about it? Do you want to court her until she's back in love with you? Do you want to call it quits? Do you want to live together as friends? There are all kinds of solutions, but without a committed love relationship, she may not be interested in a sexual relationship with you.

Does she know that you find her beautiful and sexy?
Her self-image is at a low point now, and it's up to you to make sure that she knows that you find her attractive and desirable.

She probably doesn't see herself that way anymore.

I know, for me, there were things I didn't want to be reminded of (my weight, for instance). Your wife may have her own trigger points, things that make her feel unattractive and old. She'll be much more responsive if you can help her understand that you don't see those parts of her that way.

Jesse says: I found out the hard way that menopausal women don't have a sense of humor about aging or menopause jokes, especially those told by her husband. I found myself in the doghouse a couple of times for bringing home jokes that she didn't find funny at all.

Does she have a physical barrier to a sexual relationship with you?
If she hurts when you have sex, it's going to be almost impossible to have the same kind of physical relationship that you've had before. I'm going to assume you don't want to hurt her, and I know she doesn't want to hurt. But beyond it hurting, if she's feeling exhausted because she isn't sleeping well, she may not be interested in anything that keeps her awake any extra time.

Depending on what's going on with her, there are some remedies that she might want to consider. If she's dealing with vaginal dryness, there are all kinds of lubricants available. Suggest experimenting with alternatives until she finds something that feels right to her.

Vaginal atrophy, which means that the tissues of her vagina don't stretch and may even tear with penetration, can make "traditional" sex (penetration) impossible. Sex without penetration can be pleasurable for both of you. Experiment with positions that are stimulating to you both without penetration or take turns pleasuring the other.

There are also remedies, including localized estrogen treatments and vaginal rejuvenation (a laser treatment). Just remember that it's her body – if she's not comfortable with a medical procedure or hormone therapy, don't pressure her!

If she's exhausted, then it's time to take some pressure off and help her get some sleep. Sleep issues are incredibly common. I work with almost all of my clients on sleep issues. Remedies can range from "clean sleeping habits" to melatonin supplementation to actual medical intervention (though I usually try everything before recommending she gets a sleeping aid from a doctor).

Is She Just Not that Interested in Sex These Days?

If she's experiencing a low libido (sex drive) or if she finds herself not responding to sexual stimuli, there are a couple of things that you can do together to help the situation. It begins with an agreement to allow her to control the pace and the nature of any interaction. Allowing her to feel safe and in control of how fast and how sexual things get allows her to respond with pleasure, not trepidation.

Here are three ways the two of you can begin to recreate a sexual relationship without triggering her reluctance.

Explore desire. Desire is your attraction for each other and your mutual wish to have a physical relationship. Together, play with fantasy about time spent in each other's company in romantic settings. You can play with taking turns describing a situation and then both amplifying on the scenario to add in what makes things interesting and evocative for yourselves.

Listen to what's exciting for her. Is it something you can incorporate into your own sexual play? How does it feel to you? It's just as important to notice what doesn't work for her. I know it should be "fair" and "even," but remember that the idea is to find ways to rekindle her desire for a sexual relationship.

Explore Touch. She may be unconsciously avoiding your touch because she associates it as a prelude to sex, which she's not particularly interested in right now. One way to rebuild your physical relationship is to engage in physical touch that doesn't lead to sex.

Foot rubs, shoulder rubs, or any form of touching that she enjoys are great ways to pamper her and touch her without being overtly sexual. If she's really uncomfortable with being touched, there are plenty of ways for her to experience self-pampering or pampering by another – a massage therapist, an aesthetician, a manicurist – in a way that will help her get back in touch with her body.

Explore Pleasure. Once she's ready, explore how you can create pleasure in her body. Again, this is about taking a selfless approach to the process. It's about what works for her and how she can express that to you. As you explore, ask questions. Is there a way to make it more pleasurable? Does it stop being pleasurable with more pressure, more time, more repetitions? What similar things would bring pleasure?

What About Your Performance?

If I get daily emails about enhancing my erections and dealing with erectile dysfunction as a woman, I can't imagine what it must be like to actually be a man. You must be hammered continually with the message that you can't satisfy your wife if you aren't a certain size and last a certain time frame. It must make you wonder if you're the reason she's not interested in sex anymore, that you're just not good enough.

Believe me, you are not the problem! If she's not interested in sex because it hurts, she doesn't want you to be larger or to last longer. If she's not interested because her sex drive is gone, it doesn't matter, either. And if the problem is your relationship, then you need to fix that first, and let the sexual relationship develop naturally.

I do want to mention that you are changing as well, and that can affect your sex drive. There's a similar change in hormones for men. It's called andropause and it comes from the gradual lessening of testosterone and other male hormones. And there are prostate issues. And erectile dysfunction. Honestly? I don't know a whole lot about this "guy stuff." But if these issues are getting in the way of an active and satisfying sex life, please talk to your doctor or find a good urologist. There are ways to fix this for you.

What If It All This Doesn't Fix the Problem?

I know, I know – you're hoping that doing all this will bring back your sex life. Yes, there is a chance that it won't work. Even though you've tried everything and she's been willing to experiment in hopes of rekindling her sex drive, nothing seems to be working. What can you do?

There are a couple of things that she can try if she wants things to change. There are ways to strengthen her hormonal balance through diet, exercise, and stress management. I know that can work, because it's worked for me and for many of my clients. Or she can consider hormone replacement therapy (which may not be recommended for her, depending on her medical history). Or working with a sex therapist. Or even working with a "regular" therapist. Or with a coach.

The important thing is that it's her choice. Ultimately, it's her body and her menopause. I hope she's willing to work to find solutions for what's going on, but it is her decision.

JEANNE D. ANDRUS

JESSE M. ANDRUS

Chapter 11
Some Final Thoughts

Hey, CHAMP (that's Compassionate Husband of an Amazing Menopausal Person),

In writing this book, I've attempted to open a window on the changes a woman goes through during menopause so that you, her husband, can better understand and appreciate the challenges she's facing. I've made some suggestions as to how you and she can strengthen and/or rebuild your relationship so that you can spend many more happy and productive years together.

There are a couple of things I definitely didn't do in this book.

This book wasn't designed to help a woman cope with menopause. As a menopause coach, I work with lots of women to help them design and implement their own "menopause survival plan," and it often includes how they relate to the men in their lives. (That's why I know you guys needed this book!) But that's work I do with them; this book simply provides you with some insight into what she's going through.

It also isn't a substitute for marriage counseling, relationship coaching, or sex therapy. If you and your wife need those types of services, there are many excellent providers available. (And if you can't find someone, let me know. I have several great resources to recommend to you.)

Before I leave you, I have just a couple of little topics that didn't find anywhere else to be detailed in this book so far.

Medical Treatments for Menopause

I've deliberately left out a discussion of what doctors can do to help a woman with menopause. What treatments your wife chooses for her menopause are primarily her decision. Because of her medical history, not all of them may be available to her. The following is a quick synopsis, just so you'll be familiar with the terminology.

Hormone replacement therapy (HRT). Hormones that are out of balance can sometimes be replaced with synthetic or bio-identical hormones. HRT often refers to replacement of estrogen and progesterone, but women in menopause may be dealing with replacement hormones for testosterone, thyroid hormone, or cortisol as well. HRT may not be prescribed if a woman has a history of breast cancer in the family. Topical estrogen may be prescribed for vaginal atrophy and urinary incontinence.

Antidepressants and anti-anxiety drugs. Certain drugs are prescribed to help with hot flashes as well as difficulty regulating moods. These drugs definitely carry risk of addiction and unpleasant side effects.

Hysterectomy and/or oophorectomy. These surgeries remove the uterus and cervix and the ovaries. They may be indicated for certain conditions, but represent permanent changes in her body structure. In addition, the ovaries help provide trace hormones throughout life, and there is some indication that the uterus does, too.

Vaginal rejuvenation (brand name MonaLisa Touch). A newer therapy involving laser treatment for vaginal atrophy.

I repeat: any decision about medical treatment is your wife's.

Don't Let Anyone Else Get in the Way of Your Relationship

I really hope you don't need to hear this, but I do have to say it. I'll start with my own story.

I don't tell this part of my story very often. But I want you to know, because I believe that if you're still reading, you really care about making your relationship with your wife work.

When I was in the early stages of perimenopause, I was dealing with depression and weight gain, along with some career challenges. I was also a "road warrior," a systems implementation consultant traveling four days a week, every week. Those were the strains that I (and perimenopause) put on our marriage.

Ultimately, though, that wasn't what caused our divorce. My now-ex inserted another person into our marriage. To this day, I don't know whether he had an affair. It doesn't matter. He turned to her with the problems in our marriage. He began to consider her his best friend. Her opinion was more relevant to any circumstance than mine.

In the end, he refused to put our relationship ahead of his relationship with her, and we divorced. Yes, I was jealous. And, in truth, I would expect that your wife would feel the same.

(The ever-snarky Jesse is not the person in this story. Blessedly.)

My point?

Don't turn to someone else, just because you are going through a rough time with your wife. You owe it to her, to your relationship, and to yourself (not to mention anyone you might be thinking of getting involved with) to give everything to re-igniting your relationship. You've already invested so much. And, if it really isn't going to work, you also owe it to everyone involved to finish it cleanly before moving on.

Some Further Resources for Your Wife and You

I do a lot of research about menopause, and I've summarized a lot of that research in this book. I deliberately described the changes that your wife is going through in relatively simple terms. The physiology of menopause is much more complex than I've described. I simplified it because part of letting it be her menopause is for you not to be explaining it to her.

She may want more detail or help around specific issues or symptoms. I have written several books that may help her. All are available on Amazon.com.

I Just Want to Be ME Again! *A Guide for Thriving through Menopause*
Lighten UP! *A Game Plan for Losing Weight for Women in Menopause*
Chill Out! *A Natural Guide to Controlling Hot Flashes*
Think Again! *Clearing Away the Brain Fog of Menopause*

The definitive work on what's going on in her body during menopause is *The Wisdom of Menopause* by Dr. Christiane Northrup. I use it as a reference all the time to understand specific symptoms as I help women create their own menopause survival plans.

When Googling any health issues or changes, I suggest that you and she include the word "menopause" with the symptom. Otherwise, you may fall into the "weird, scary disease" trap, where the results are full of "answers" that terrify you both.

On the subject of andropause, the male analogue to menopause, there's less available than I'd like to see. Much of it centers on testosterone replacement. As with hormone replacement therapy, testosterone replacement is a personal decision. One of the better books I found while searching for decent sources is *Andropause: The Complete Male Menopause Guide* by Brady Howard.

Want more? My website, www.menopause.guru, is where I write and post about menopause. And I love connecting with women and their men about what is going on in their lives and anything they've found to make it better.

JEANNE D. ANDRUS
84 JESSE M. ANDRUS

Hey, Can I Talk to Your Wife for a Minute?

Pssst! Is he gone?

Good. Cuz this is just between us women.

In the years I've been working with women, I find that one of the most common questions I get asked is "How do I explain this to my husband?"

So, I created this book.

Most of the time, I find that you've read it before you give it to him, because, if you're like me, you don't want him making things worse by explaining to you what your body is doing(!), or trying to fix you, or trying to take over the whole thing. (You might even tear out this page!)

In telling him NOT to do those things, and HOW to find out exactly what support you need at this time in your life, I hope I've helped open up the lines of communication between you two. And in that communication window, you have the opportunity to work with him to redesign your relationship for this next phase of your lives. I know that revisiting "the rules" of your relationship can really rekindle the love between you.

And if you need more detailed information about what's happening in your body and how you can survive menopause and live your best life yet, I've written that book, too. It goes deeper into the changes that you're going through.

Even more importantly, it helps you find some relief from the symptoms that you may be experiencing.

And I'd love to send you a pdf copy of the book. Just go to http://menopause.guru/free-book and tell me where to send it. (It's called *"I Just Want to be ME Again!"*).

Here's to you, beautiful!

Jeanne

Acknowledgments

When I started this journey into writing a little over two years ago, I had no idea how rapidly it would grow from one book to five. That it did is not due so much to my own writing ability, but to the community that has supported and encouraged me. There are so many to thank that I'm sure I'll forget someone.

First of all, thanks to Angela Lauria and Difference Press, and especially, but not limited to my editors, Grace Kerina and Maggie McReynolds. You make me sound better than I could ever sound without you. To the support team at Difference Press, Paul Brycock and the entire support staff, thank you for always welcoming me, in whatever castle we find ourselves.

Thanks to Sharon Pope, whose leadership in the field of relationship coaching has been a source of inspiration to me, and specifically, for providing a delightful foreword to this work. Should your (the reader's) relationship need fine-tuning or a major overhaul, I can think of no one better to recommend to you than Sharon! (www.sharonpopetruth.com)

Thanks, too, to all my clients, especially the ones who have allowed me to share parts of their stories here and in my previous books. You've taught me much in your willingness to be vulnerable and to grow into the amazing women you've become. Thank you for allowing me to be part of your journey.

To my coaches and friends who have encouraged my research and my coaching, many thanks. To the "Girlfriends," the "Enchanted Circle," and the "Order of the Plume," you make me want to do better. To the five Difference Press "cohorts" I've been privileged to work with, thank you for dozens of insightful reads. To Cassie, Rosslyn, and Darryl, thank you for leading me to many insights into myself, without which this book would not be possible. And to Jill (Not Your Average

Running Coach) for helping me to literally run away from my problems again!

To my family, especially Jesse, Jamie, Kate, and Miles, thank you for the unwavering support, even when my writing meant I was less present than I should have been in our family life. To my fur family – Sweetie, Harry, and Dora – thank you for listening to me mutter, mumble, and whine as I tried to find just the right word.

Out in the world, there are voices that have influenced my thinking, helped me understand the gift of menopause, and learn to articulate the truth that bloomed first in my own heart before finding their words in the world of facts. Without them, I wouldn't have ever affected my own healing, nor been able to help in the healing of my clients. Their work has been the backbone of mine, not just in this book, but in every word I write and speak, and with every client I coach.

Dr. Christiane Northrup and Dr. Louanne Brizendine, you've both inspired me and informed me with your work, which helps explain why "The Change" changes everything. Without your insights, it would have been impossible to realize how wide the doors open to us as menopause changes us.

To the pioneers of the Low Carb world who have tirelessly fought against the "fat makes you fat" fallacy – Dr. Robert Atkins, Jonny Bowden, Loren Cordain, and so many more – thank you for changing the way the world thinks about eating, and for providing the science that proves it. And to Dr. Kathryn Vargo, who, when I asked about Atkins, convinced me to give it a try.

To Gay Hendricks, whom I first encountered in The Big Leap, for the words of wisdom that underlie this book. After a dozen road trips spent listening to Learning to Love Yourself, I think I'm finally getting it.

To the countless researchers in the field of endocrinology who publish and synopsize their work on the Internet, thank you for selflessly spreading your knowledge and the fruits of your labors.

And finally, once again, I must thank Rich, without whom I wouldn't have the deep, visceral understanding of just why it is so important that both women and men understand the changes that happen to a woman during menopause and that couples communicate throughout.

JEANNE D. ANDRUS
JESSE M. ANDRUS

About The Authors

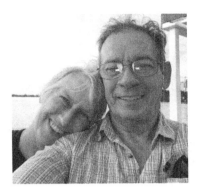

Jeanne and Jesse Andrus met while kayaking the whitewater Coosa River, shortly after Jeanne moved to Alabama following her divorce from her first husband. They were married in 2011 on the bluff overlooking their favorite rapid on that river. They make their home on the Northshore of Lake Pontchartrain, in the Greater New Orleans region.

At the age of 54, Jeanne Andrus left the corporate world to pursue her passion - helping women struggling with menopause recapture their health, fitness, and zest for life. She's been doing this research and work for a decade now.

Jeanne is the author of five international bestsellers and has spoken in the United States and Europe about the impacts of menopause and how women can recapture their best selves during their Menopause Journey.

For her most recent work, she enlisted Jesse's help to explain the man's point of view and ask the questions that formed the basis of Where Is My Wife and What Have You Done with Her? She says his sense of humor has been instrumental in injecting a sense of fun into the important subject of maintaining the relationship between husband and wife as midlife changes them.

JEANNE D. ANDRUS

JESSE M. ANDRUS

Other Books From
The Menopause Guru

I Just Want to Be ME, Again! (Nov. 2015)

"Upon the recommendation of a wise and kind friend, I read this book in spite of my state of denial. It turns out that "I Just Want To Be Me Again" is just as useful for those of us nearing perimenopause as it is for those already in the throes of menopause. In fact, it might even be MORE useful at that point because a little advanced planning can help prevent and/or lighten certain challenges."

Lighten Up! (Mar. 2016)

"A weight loss book with a couple of great twists. First, it's designed specifically for women whose bodies are dealing with the changes of menopause. That's great, because too many so-called experts deny there's anything different about it (and we all know there is). And, second, she focuses on what she calls the "Inner Game" of weight loss and lightening up - getting in touch with ourselves and our needs."

Chill Out! (Sept. 2016)

"Chill Out! By Jeanne Andrus is a timely read for me because everyone keeps asking me if I have reached menopause yet... Her step by step approach to dealing with the often miserable parts of menopause is sensible and easy to implement."

Think Again! (Nov. 2016)

"Rather than treating menopause as a time of life to "suffer through," Jeanne helps us look for the gifts and wisdom in the symptoms and experiences that show up, blended with science and practical steps to take to feel supported and to thrive.

Made in the USA
Monee, IL
17 May 2023

33906359R00066